I0705101

Science nutritional of the spirulina

Cesar Gonzalez Andrade

Science nutritional of the spirulina

Learn about the science-proven benefits of spirulina.

Cesar Gonzalez Andrade

Warning

Health sciences such as nutrition are a constantly changing field and therefore the information contained herein may vary. This book is of an informative nature and the information presented should not be taken as a substitute for a prescription, diagnosis, or medical treatment. The author is not responsible for the damages caused by omitting this warning. It is always recommended to consult a doctor or nutritionist.

Index

Preface 1

Gratitude 4

Introducción 5

   Lipids 7

      Triglycerides 7

      Cholesterol 8

      Low-density lipoprotein 8

      High-density lipoprotein 9

   Hypertension 9

   Antioxidant 10

   Exercise 10

      Oxygen consumption 11

      Protein 11

      Improved results 12

   Immune system 12

   Human immunodeficiency virus 13

   Supplementation for Children.................. 14

Conclusions 15

Bibliography 16

Preface

We all seek to solve our health problems with reliable information, in a more natural way and without resorting to medications or surgeries, however, the information we find on the internet is often confusing, contradictory, wrong or dangerous, and does not solve our problems.

We also have the information that we can find in books, however, here we have another problem, the books that are available are usually of two types: the first is a book easy to read and understand, but with unreliable information that comes from opinions and not from research, the second is a book with accurate and scientific information but difficult to read, with many technicalities and few or no practical recommendations.

Therefore, in this book you will find the best of both types of books:

The information presented in this book was obtained from scientific research articles published in indexed scientific journals, they are the most reliable source in terms of health issues. With this information you can take actions to improve your health and with better results.

In all scientific articles a very technical language is used, with very complex figures and formulas, explaining the methodology that was used, and the results are usually explained statistically, but in this book you will find the information of the results and their conclusions in a much clearer and above all practical way, so that you can use it for your benefit.

The articles reviewed and cited in this book are the publications of researchers with PhD or Postdoctoral degrees in the subject of this publication. For these articles to be published in indexed journals they must be reviewed by other expert researchers in the field, to confirm that their results are correct.

Throughout the book at the end of certain sentences or paragraphs you will find superscripts like this: ([1]), this statement can be used to find in the bibliography the scientific article from which the cited information was obtained. In addition, you will find in italics the scientific name of the species to be able to differentiate it from the rest of the text.

There are diverse types of research, such as in vitro assays, which focus on studying cells or microorganisms; there is also observational research, where only the facts that the researcher observes first-hand without performing any intervention are described. However, for this book most of the research that was consulted were human clinical trials and randomized controlled trials. The results of randomized controlled trials in humans are considered the most accurate and dependable in health.

The author César González Andrade studied the degree in Nutrition at the Faculty of Nutrition of the Autonomous University of the State of Morelos, he is the author of the nutrition books:

The Nutritional Science of Teas.

Habits and Nutrition Against Baldness.

Gratitude

Thanks to the people who bought this book to learn about nutrition and improve their health, that of their family or that of someone who needs it.

If you like the content of the book, you can leave comments, topic suggestions and rate this book on Amazon, that will help me a lot so that more people know about my publications and continue to produce books on interesting and useful nutrition topics.

Remember that many problems can be prevented or treated with a correct diet.

Introducción

Spirulina is a cyanobacterium that is currently used as a food supplement worldwide. Cyanobacteria are also known as green algae and are found in all waters of the world. There are two specific species of cyanobacteria that are defined as spirulina *Arthrospira platensis* and *Arthrospira maxima*, both species have been widely studied and usually food supplements one or both.

It is normally consumed as a dehydrated supplement in various presentations such as pills, capsules or powder and is dark green in color. Dehydration of food involves removing as much water as possible, and spirulina has 95 percent water naturally.

Half the weight of spirulina when dehydrated is protein, this means that 100 grams of spirulina contribute 50 grams to the diet, while beef provides 30 grams of protein on average. In addition, it contains calcium, phosphorus, magnesium, iron, and potassium, due to this amount of nutrients many people around the world consider it a superfood[1].

However, sometimes spirulina is attributed properties and benefits that are not proven or simply not true, in addition there is a group of people who should not consume spirulina. Therefore, this book will present the main results of clinical trials in humans, which prove

the benefits of consuming spirulina as a food supplement.

Lipids

Lipids can be fats or oils, fats are kept in a solid state at room temperature, and oils are kept in a liquid state. Lipids are found in the membranes of cells and are especially important for the proper functioning of the human body. Another important function of lipids is to store energy in the form of triglycerides in adipose tissue. A person who is overweight or obese usually has an excess of adipose tissue under the skin, in the abdomen and torso of the body.

Some of the most important lipids for the human body are lipoproteins, cholesterol, and triglycerides.[2]

Triglycerides

Triglycerides are lipids or fats that function in our body as energy storage, normally found in our body within adipocytes, which are the cells found in adipose tissue under the skin.

Normal triglyceride levels are less than 150 milligrams per deciliter, but high triglyceride levels are associated with diseases such as hypertension and cardiovascular disease.[3]

Spirulina is particularly good for reducing blood triglyceride levels, it can decrease between 50 and 100 milligrams per deciliter in the blood, without exercising or modifying the diet. The reduction of blood triglycerides can be reached at 6 weeks after consuming 4.5 grams of spirulina a day.[4]

Cholesterol

Cholesterol is a lipid found in lipoproteins, and in cell membranes. Healthy cholesterol levels are less than 200 milligrams per deciliter. While high cholesterol levels are called hypercholesterolemia and are associated with diseases such as hypertension and atherosclerotic cardiovascular disease.[5,6]

Consuming spirulina can reduce 20 milligrams over deciliter in blood cholesterol levels, after 6 weeks consuming 4.5 grams of spirulina a day.[4]

Low-density lipoprotein

It is a lipid that serves to transport cholesterol throughout the human body, it is known as low-density lipoprotein (LDL) because it contains few proteins. It is recommended to have a level less than 100 milligrams per deciliter in blood.[5,7]

Spirulina is particularly good at reducing low-density lipoprotein levels, it can decrease 20 milligrams per deciliter in the blood in just six weeks consuming 4.5 grams daily.[4]

High-density lipoprotein

It is a lipid that serves to transport other lipids such as cholesterol through the human body, it is known as high-density lipoprotein (HDL) because it is made up of more proteins than lipids. It is recommended to have between 40 to 60 milligrams per deciliter in blood. Below 40 milligrams people can develop atherosclerosis.[5,8]

Spirulina can reduce levels of cholesterol, triglycerides and low-density lipoprotein that are bad lipids for health, and, in addition, it can increase levels of high-density lipoproteins that are good for the human body. Daily consumption of 4.5 grams of spirulina can increase 7 milligrams per deciliter of high-density lipoproteins in the blood.[4]

Hypertension

Hypertension is systolic blood pressure of 130 or higher and diastolic blood pressure greater than 80. It is one of the most common chronic diseases today. It is associated with strokes, myocardial infarctions, heart failure and kidney failure[9]

Daily consumption of 4.5 grams of spirulina for 6 weeks can reduce systolic blood pressure by 130 to 110 and diastolic blood pressure by 80 to 70. It also helps decrease damage to the arteries by free radicals and prevents inflammation of the blood vessels.[410]

Antioxidant

Antioxidants are small organic molecules that decrease free radical damage to the cells and tissues of the human body. Free radicals are formed naturally within the human body by metabolism.[11]

An increase in free radicals is associated with chronic inflammation, and can be harmful in people with obesity, diabetes, atherosclerosis, and cancer.[11]

Exercise

Normally our body is in a state of rest, however, when performing an exercise, a greater physical, metabolic, respiratory, and cardiovascular effort is required. To adapt to this effort the body must improve its physical condition, metabolic pathways, respiratory capacity, and the ability to transport blood with oxygen throughout the body. It is for this reason that exercise improves our health.[12]

Oxygen consumption

A patient's cardiopulmonary function can be assessed with maximum oxygen uptake. Therefore, the higher the oxygen consumption, the better the health of the heart and lungs, in addition, it improves performance in sports avoiding fatigue of the muscles.[13]

Consuming 4.5 grams of spirulina for 6 weeks increases the maximum volume of oxygen used when a person performs high-intensity exercises such as short runs and increases the time it takes to become fatigued.[14]

In addition, the consumption of spirulina also increases hemoglobin levels in the blood and improves oxygen utilization, for these reasons spirulina also benefits athletes who perform prolonged exercises.[15]

Protein

Proteins are organic molecules that make up cells, tissues, organs, and the human body. For this reason, you should increase your consumption to increase muscle mass with physical exercise. They are usually found in foods of animal origin such as meats, eggs, or milk.[16]

Improved results

The results of exercise can be measured in two ways, by reducing human body fat and increasing muscle mass. And at the same time these results can be achieved by modifying the amount of exercise or modifying the diet.[17]

In one study two groups of people performed the same amount of exercise for 6 weeks, but one group consumed 4.5 grams of spirulina every day and the other group did not consume spirulina. The group that consumed spirulina lost on average 2.2 kilograms, while the group of people who did not consume spirulina only lost 1.6 kilograms. In addition, consuming spirulina reduces appetite.[1418]

Immune system

The immune system is responsible for preventing the infection of the human body by pathogens such as bacteria, viruses, and fungi. It consists of physical barriers such as skin, saliva, tears, and mucus; and it is also composed of cells specialized in eliminating pathogens when they are already inside the human body.[19]

Human immunodeficiency virus

It is a virus that is transmitted sexually or by blood transfusion. It eliminates CD4+ T cells and causes a poor immune response, so any virus, bacteria or fungus can infect the human body.[20]

The human immunodeficiency virus causes alterations in glucose metabolism that can generate diabetes in patients. However, consuming spirulina for 8 weeks increases insulin sensitivity, reducing blood glucose levels, which reduces the chance of developing diabetes.[21]

People who have the human immunodeficiency virus also develop alterations in lipid metabolism such as cholesterol or elevated triglycerides, decreased high-density lipoprotein. The consumption of spirulina for 6 months decreases these alterations in lipid metabolism.[22]

Consuming spirulina for 12 months increases the CD4 cells of the immune system and decreases the viral load within the human body. It also works as a specific

antioxidant for people who have the human immunodeficiency virus.[23][24]

Supplementation for Children

Cognitive development during early childhood is especially important for children, it is during this stage that
the frontal lobe matures, memory develops, planning
actions or the appearance of thought and permanence
of the object. For a child to develop properly, he must
consume a correct amount of protein and avoid malnutrition.[25]

Child malnutrition is a global problem. However, consuming 10 grams of spirulina as a dietary supplement
increases 5 grams of protein to the children's diet.[26]

Conclusions

To get most of the benefits, scientific research suggests consuming more than 2 grams of spirulina for more than 6 weeks. People who have obesity, cholesterol and high triglycerides are the ones who get the most benefits from consuming spirulina. In addition, better results are obtained when exercising at least 3 times a week.[2728]

The consumption of spirulina is considered safe. However, it can also decrease blood iron levels and therefore would not be recommended for people who have anemia.[1029]

Bibliography